Stay In the Game: Pickleball for Seniors

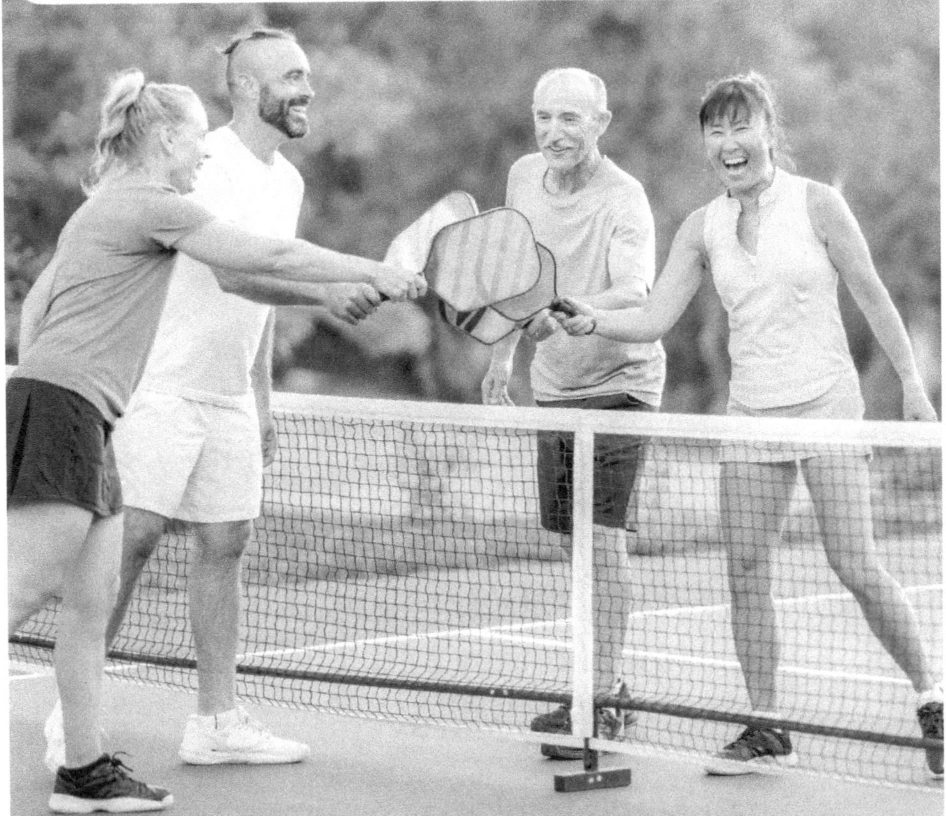

By David & Deb Jeffrey

Large Print

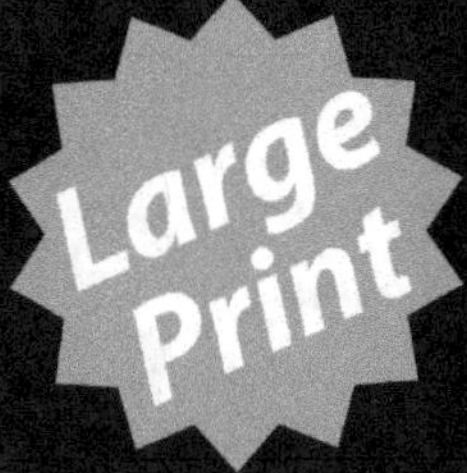

Tailored advice on preventing and managing common injuries for mature players,

WITH BONUS PICKLEBALL LOG

For other Pickleball themed publications and products, please scan the QR code, or visit www.debjeffrey.com/pickleball

Stay In The Game: Pickleball for Seniors
ISBN: 9798326178398

Stay In The Game: Pickleball For Seniors

Tailored advice on preventing and managing common injuries for mature players. From warm-up techniques to proactive exercises, this concise guide equips seniors with the knowledge to stay safe, healthy, and thriving on the court, ensuring a sustained love for the game.

By
David & Deb Jeffrey

INTRO

 My wife and I love to play pickleball. It's a great sport, and a wonderful way to meet and interact with like-minded people, get some exercise, and have some fun in the sun.

After playing pickleball for several years, I have met many seniors who are either playing injured or are playing in such a way that there is an injury just waiting to happen. As a lifelong athlete, former tennis instructor, and licensed Occupational Therapist, specializing in Ergonomics, Hand & Upper Extremities, my goal is to share information that will help you play the game smarter, safer and longer. And if you are contemplating the sport and you have an injury or medical condition that you are concerned about, this book shares some things to consider before getting out on the court. This is important to me because as a therapist for over 35 years, I have been blessed to work with neurology, pulmonary, and cardiac patients of all ages. And having suffered a stroke myself, which initially resulted in total left sided paralysis, I made a complete recovery which enabled me to resume teaching tennis and engage in a wide variety of other competitive sports. Our bodies have amazing abilities to overcome many physical, visual and emotional setbacks allowing us to enjoy returning to playing a variety of sports and engaging in activities that restore our joy and sense of well-being.

Pickleball is more than just hitting a ball with a paddle. It requires training in HOW to hit a variety of shots, correctly, to help reduce the force loads, (stress/strain), that are placed on the joints of your thumb, fingers, wrist, elbow, and shoulder. Hitting shots incorrectly can increase the force loads on the joints and may result in overuse injuries.

In addition to the upper body considerations, it is important to consider your lower body function, including standing balance, your ability to move forward, sideways, diagonally and backwards, and transitioning from walking, jogging, sprinting, lunging, stepping, bending and stretching. These movements place significant force loads on the fascia, (a layer of connective tissue below the skin that supports muscles, organs, and bones), as well as the covering on the bottom of your feet, which can result in fascial tears, swelling and pain. Another cause of fascial tears is wearing poorly fitting shoes, and failure to wear proper insoles.

TIP: I wear SLO Motion insoles, but you may receive help from visiting your podiatrist and trying on a variety of products, walking and jogging in them before buying an insole.

It is at this point that I need to stress that if you are having pain or weakness, visit your doctor and ask for a consultation with a physical or occupational therapist, so that they can evaluate your need for supportive straps, splints, joint wraps, training in the use of Kinesio Tape applications, and anti-inflammatory gels and spray-on pain relief medications.

NOTE: Please check with your physician or specialist before engaging in the sport of Pickleball or carrying out any of the information contained in this book.

Let's start with two big questions that you may have...

Could I play pickleball?

You may be asking this question because you have seen how much fun pickleball players seem to have while playing the sport, but you may question your ability to learn and play pickleball at your age, or with your medical, physical or visual issues.

Pickleball is played at various levels, from beginner (level 1.0) to expert (level 5.5), based on the USA Pickleball ratings scale.

While it is exciting to watch pickleball players who have refined their abilities to skillfully play the game, I encourage you to observe novice players whose skill levels are at the 1.0-2.5 level. These players are learning the rules and game etiquette and will give you a clue as to what upper and lower body coordination, strength and endurance will be needed to engage in the sport.

As I stated previously, I am an Occupational, Ergonomic and Hand Therapist, with training in Cardiac and Pulmonary Rehabilitation programs at multiple hospitals. Persons who have these medical issues often can regain the physiological abilities to engage in controlled levels of cardiac and pulmonary demands during exercise and functional activity. For persons with diagnosed cardiac and pulmonary issues, it is essential to meet with your cardiologist and pulmonologist, to seek their advice and approval to start playing pickleball. And, if you do have any preexisting-existing conditions, it is strongly encouraged that you wear or carry medical alert information, so that if you are involved in an emergency situation, first responders and your medical care team can treat you quickly and appropriately, according to your stated needs. It is also possible that you could be fitted with cardiac monitor and/or pulmonary pulse oximeter to ensure that your cardio/pulmonary vitals are staying within your physician's stated parameters. These monitors will help you know when you need a break based upon your physician's designated parameters. It would be wise to discuss your potential need for these devices and activity questions with your physician. Remember that the above-mentioned devices are medical tools that enable you to enjoy playing pickleball at a level of activity safe for you. They are wrongly perceived as a ball and chain, preventing you from enjoying exercising.

Should I play pickleball?

The answer to this question extends beyond cardio and pulmonary issues. Repetitive overuse issues such as pickleball elbow, rotator cuff injuries, carpal tunnel syndrome, and others can occur.

Pickleball elbow, (lateral epicondylitis), presents as pain, soreness and weakness that can radiate from the elbow to the forearm and wrist. It can be treated by resting and icing (to reduce swelling) and improving your shot mechanics; But it is recommended that you see your doctor and ask for an occupational or physical therapy consult to evaluate and treat any existing therapeutic concerns.

Rotator cuff injuries are common and cause

pain, weakness, and limited mobility in the affected shoulder, and should be evaluated by your physician.

Carpal tunnel syndrome is another common injury that can result from excessive pressure on the median nerve distribution to aspects of the hand and wrist, resulting in numbness, tingling and burning pain at the wrist and fingers. Left untreated functional use of the affected hand will result in significant impairment.

Carpal Tunnel symptoms can often be resolved with median nerve gliding exercises, anti-inflammatory medication injections into the carpal tunnel, as well as stabilizing of the wrist with functional hand and wrist splints and nighttime use of compression gloves to control edema. I struggled with this issue for years, but because of faithfully performing the above-mentioned treatment, my wrist is typically pain free while playing pickleball and engaging in functional tasks of daily living. Surgical release of the fascia at the carpal tunnel is highly effective in freeing the median nerve and restoring hand function.

The hallmark exercise for reducing carpal tunnel symptoms is *Median Nerve Gliding*. This exercise stretches the Palmer Fascia (Protective covering over the fingers and palm of the hand). This maneuver decreases pressure from the fascia upon the median nerve, resulting in less pain and swelling while restoring active movement and grip strength.

Median Nerve Gliding Exercise -

STEP 1

Start with the fingers in a loose fist, with the thumb flexed or bent over the fingers. Hold for 5-10 seconds).

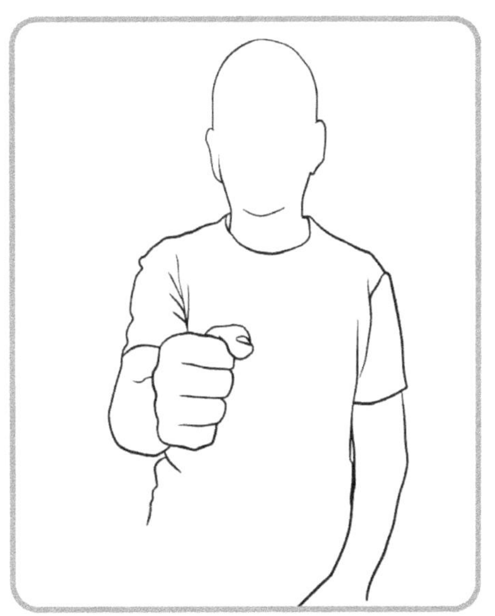

STEP 2

Extend your thumb and fingers to full extension simultaneously.

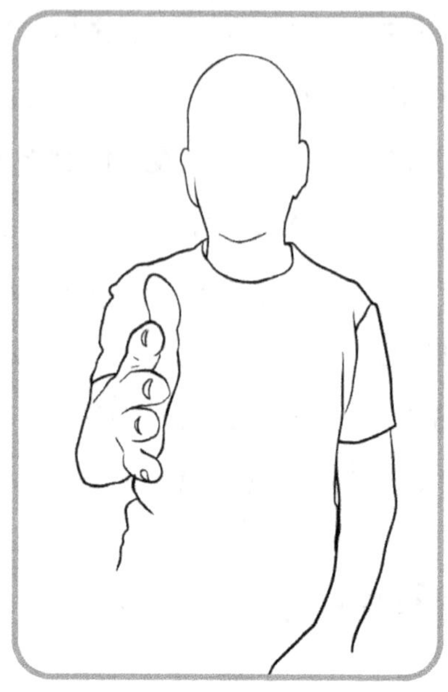

STEP 3

Turn your palm up.

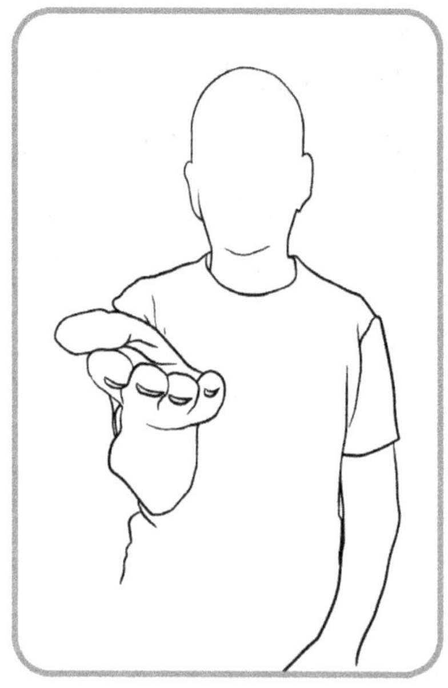

STEP 4

Extend your wrist, so that your fingers are angled towards the ground.

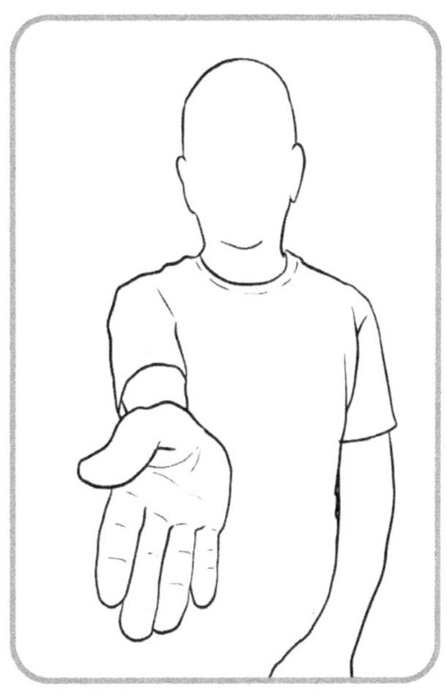

STEP 5

Extend your thumb, away from your fingers.

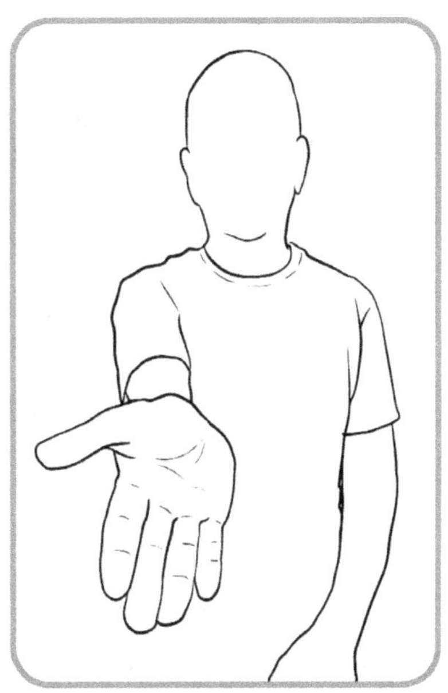

STEP 6

Gently grab and hold of your thumb with your opposite hand, while extending your elbow fully; gradually and gently pull the thumb away from the fingers using it as an assist to extend your wrist as far as is tolerable.

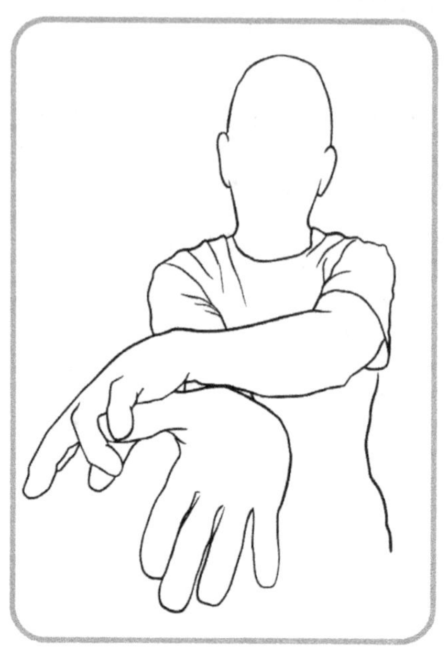

Hold for 30-60 seconds. Perform a total of 5-10 repetitions; 2-3 times per day, or as tolerated.

This exercise will stretch all fingers and wrist tendons. Increasing extension in this manner improves finger and wrist mobility while lengthening tendons and gliding the median nerve resulting in increased joint range of motion, decreased pain and increased ability to play pickleball for extended time with significantly improved hand strength and gripping control.

STEP 7

Ice. Using a large bowl, fill it with water to half-full and add four to five ice cubes.

With your hand open, submerge the affected hand into the water for 5-10 seconds.

Remove for 20 seconds, then repeat for 3-5 repetitions as is tolerable.

NOTE: if the pain becomes too intense remove your hand from the water and wrap it in a warm towel until the pain is manageable. Slowly introduce this technique into your pain management program. Icing might aggravate symptoms if you have a history of cardiac disease, seizures, peripheral neuropathy, severe neuropathy, severe arthritis and other Vaso constricting issues, so be sure to obtain your physician's approval prior to trying median nerve gliding and icing.

Another key part of reducing pressure on the median nerve at the wrist is to **build up the diameter of the Pickleball paddle grip**. This can be done by getting some pickleball paddle grip tape and wrapping the handle of your Pickleball paddle, to increase the diameter of the grip, which reduces load force while gripping and playing Pickleball. The best fit is to apply enough of the grip tape to increase the handle diameter so that when gripping the handle your fingertips are separated from your thumb, (while gripping your paddle by the width of your middle finger of your other hand). This will give you good paddle control and reduce hand and wrist discomfort.

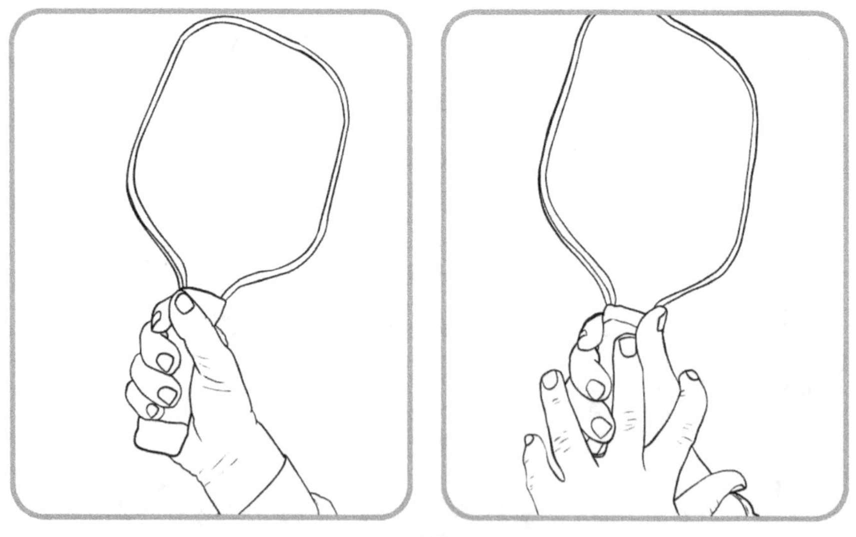

I encourage you to **keep a written journal** of your Pickleball play, to figure out how much time you can play before you need to take a break to perform wrist stretching. Also, you can find weightlifting gloves that have metal stays in the palmer aspect of the wrist, ending at mid palm. Wearing these while playing Pickleball gives excellent extended relief, for prolonging your Pickleball playing time.

If you are experiencing weakness and joint discomfort in your fingers, you can try **buddy-taping** two adjacent fingers to strengthen fingers and reduce joint discomfort. You can use Kinesio Tape, flexible athletic tape, or buddy taping splints.

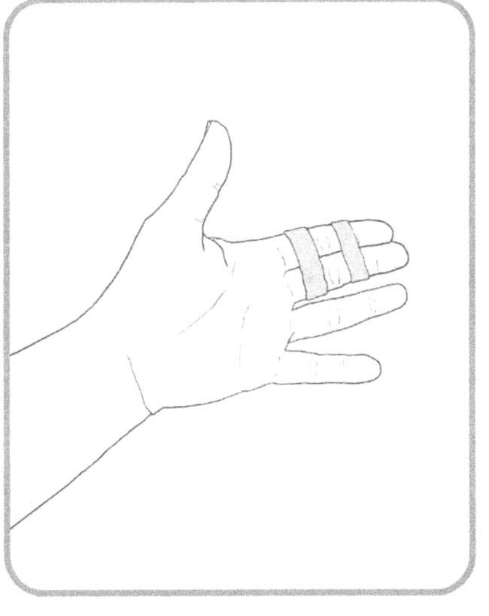

Note: Kinesio tape can also be used on thumbs, wrists, elbows, knees, ankles, foot arches, etc. See manufacturer application guidelines.

If you need to statbilize or maintain joint integrity, your therapist might suggest **Thermo-plastic splints**. Thermo-plastic splints can be molded by a therapist for wrist, fingers and ankles. These splints are held in place by flexible bands. They stabilize the affected joints, maintaining joint integrity, while keeping pain under control.

Flexible splints - Flexible splints and braces can be found Online at Amazon.com. Ask your Occupational Therapist for upper extremity splints (hand, wrist, elbow), and your Physical Therapist for shoulder, back, knee and ankle splints and braces. These consultations are essential to learn splint application and fitting guidelines, as well as wearing duration and follow-up therapy management, such as icing, pain control gels, and use of night splints to protect the joints while you are resting or sleeping.

Some people with arthritis of the MP joints or carpal tunnel syndrome might find **night-time wrist extension splints and braces** uncomfortable, so they disregard them, preventing the essential need to stretch wrist tendons and muscles into prolonged static extension.

I so appreciate the advice of Arthur Ashe, to "Start where you are, use what you have, and do what you can." We will take this advice and use what you have, a standard pillow and washcloth or hand towel, to help facilitate wrist mobility, decrease flexion contracture, and improve hand and wrist function.

Pillow with pillowcase – Slip your hand under the pillowcase and wrap your fingers around the end of the pillow, to maintain wrist extension.

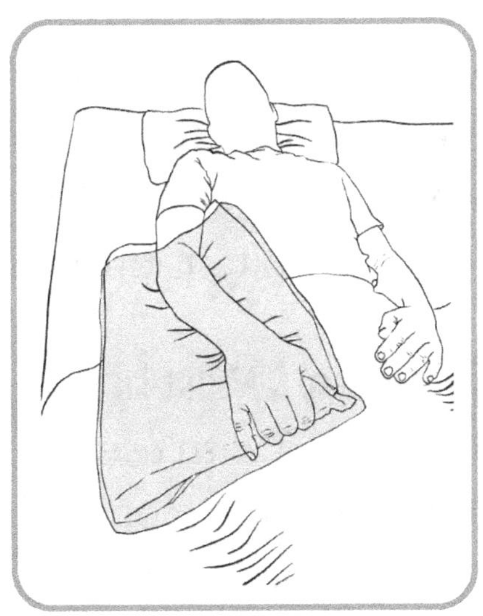

Wash cloth or hand towel – Roll up the washcloth or hand towel and secure with rubber

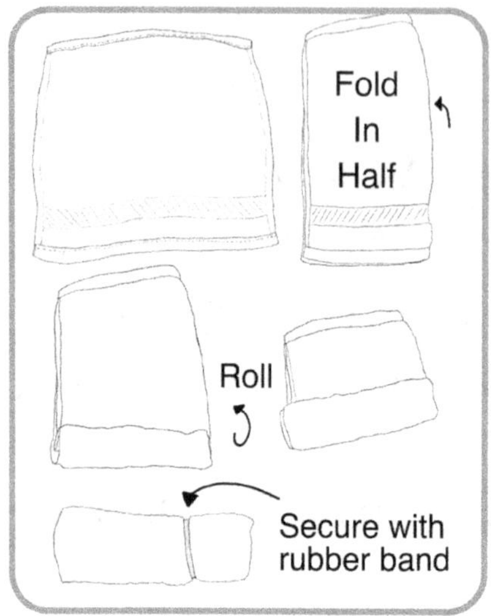

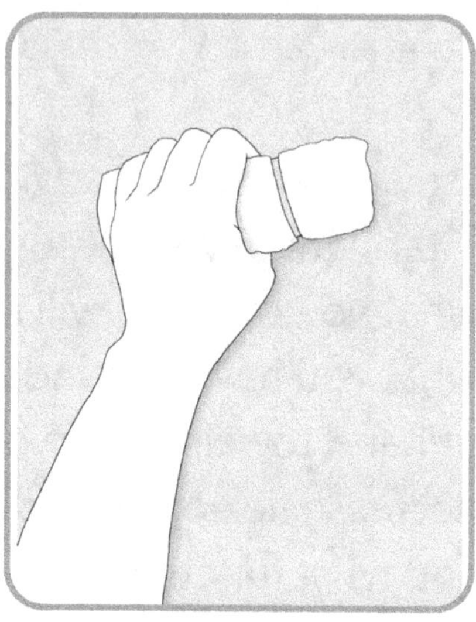

bands, to hold the shape. Then simply place your hand around the "roll", a comfortable, pain free way to stretch the hand and wrist tendons into 20°-30° of extension while you sleep.

Summary - Most hand and wrist issues can be reduced with use of a variety of anti-inflammatories, coupled with median nerve gliding exercise, icing and wearing flexible wrist support when playing pickleball. Wearing static splints at night while sleeping also reduces nerve impingement, resulting in decreased pain.

I thank you for your time and the opportunity to share some therapy techniques with you. Please consult with your physician prior to implementing any of these recommendations.

Now, I'd like to introduce my wife Deb. She will be sharing more practical tips and information for dealing with lower body aches, pains and injuries.

God bless you and enjoy playing pickleball.

David Jeffrey, OTR/L/Hand Therapist

SECTION 2

Hi, I'm David's wife Deb. Unlike David, I am not a lifelong athlete. I am what you might call a casual athlete - one who goes on leisurely bike rides, hikes, and when I play pickleball, it is for socialization and fun.

Not being super athletic, my body hasn't been quite as forgiving as David's, so while he is observing people with injuries, I have had my share of injuries including: extensor hood tear with repair and tendon transfer in my dominant hand; broken ankle; hip labrum tear and repair; displaced cartilage in my patella;

and spondylolisthesis and severe stenosis of the spine. All the injuries have resulted in hours of occupational and physical therapy, and since I am a lifelong learner, I asked a lot of questions and would like to share what I've learned along the way.

SHOES...

My physical therapist asked which shoes I wore to play pickleball. I was wearing court shoes, which was a good thing because they were designed for the task and to provide the proper support. However, as he "evaluated" my shoes, he shared these observations:

They were too worn. I think his exact words were, "You are one pickleball slide away from going through the soles of those shoes." The takeaway -- be sure your shoes have adequate tread on them.

In response to my question about knee pain when playing, he checked three specific areas and made these comments:

First, my shoelaces. He asked if I slipped my shoes on and off without tying them. I don't, but I hate it when my feet get hot, so I purposefully hadn't been tying my shoes very securely. He said that this was a problem because my arch wasn't properly supported. He said that the arch support in the shoe could only do its job if the shoe was tied correctly.

He then explained HOW to tie my shoes for best support:

STEP 1

Place your foot in your shoe and curl your toes down. Keep them curled down as you tighten your laces, pulling taught the lace on the inside of the foot.

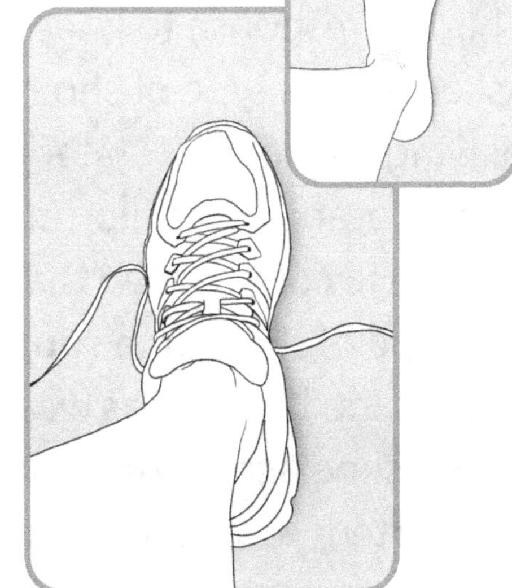

STEP 2

Then when your laces are secure, uncurl your toes and lift the toe of your shoe off the ground to tie the laces at the ankle.

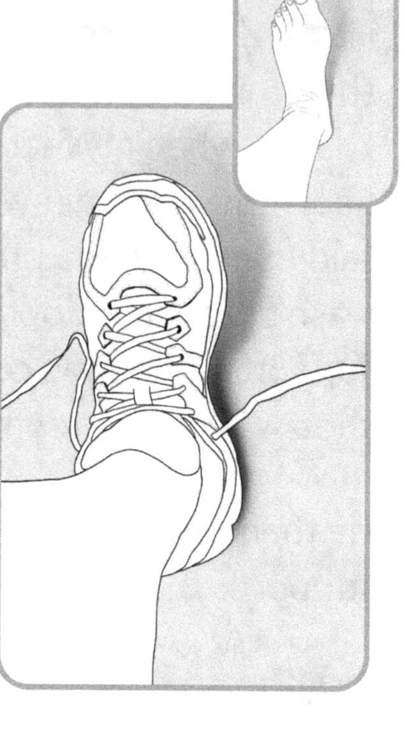

Second, he evaluated my hips and noted that my right leg is ever so slightly longer than my left and suggested a small lift be placed in the heel of my left shoe, to balance out my body.

Third, in response to knee pain in general, he asked for the type of shoes I wore when not playing pickleball. I stated that I go barefoot at home, and wear slip-ons when I must wear shoes. He commented that regardless of the type of shoe, arch support is particularly important, because as was said in the comment about shoelaces, when your arch isn't properly supported, your arch collapses, which puts more pressure on the inside of your knee, which can result in knee pain and potential injury.

In regards to knee pain, mine was helped by the above, but an orthopedic surgeon friend of ours mentioned that other common knee pain problems can be caused by miniscus tears or arthritis, so be sure to discuss your knee pain with your doctor for a proper diagnosis.

HIP PAIN:

In the song, *Dem Bones*, we all learned that, "The thigh bone's connected to the hip bone", and, "The hip bone's connected to the backbone." Well, my physical therapist shared the importance of supporting your backbone (spine) with a strong core.

There are a number of core strengthening exercise options, but because your back is involved, please be sure that whatever exercises you incorporate into your core strengthening routine, they are approved by your doctor or therapist.

So why am I talking about the core when the topic is hip pain? Because when our core is weak, we tend to adapt by standing, sitting and moving in ways that can ultimately cause other parts of our body to become out of alignment, or experience pain. This is what was happening with my hip. My core was weak, which resulted in poor posture and my body being out of alignment, with my hip feeling the pain.

One thing my therapist suggested while playing pickleball was to try using a SI Belt (Sacroiliac belt). It is an elastic support, similar to a back support, but narrower and is worn around the hips and pelvis. I tried it and it provided just enough support to allow me to play pain-free. Of course, the use the of a SI Belt was only suggested by my therapist as a band-aid, with the ultimate focus being on strengthening the core muscles.

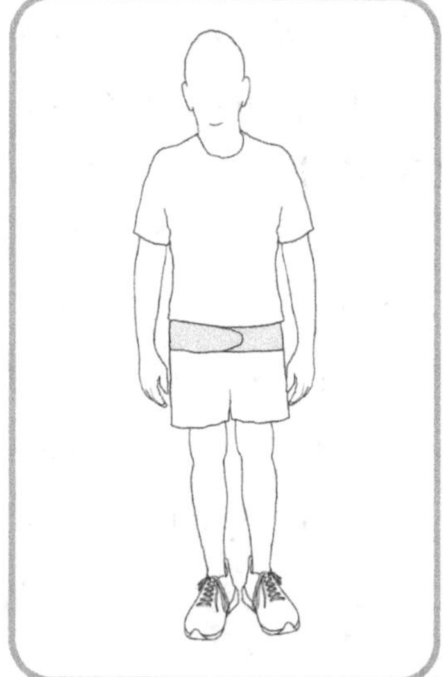

WARM UP

Given my knee, hip and back issues, I asked for pickleball warm-up advice. This is what my physical therapist suggested:

First, an observation that he made. He noticed that many people do arm circles and waist twists to warm up the upper body, but totally neglect their lower body. The core and lower body are what hold you up and move you about the court, so warming up these parts of the body is vital to helping to keep you safe and prepared for playing pickleball.

Don't warm up with slow stretches. Instead, do more dynamic movements. Why? Because they will gradually increase the heart rate and blood flow and help prepare your body for better and safer movement on the court.

Warm-up routine:

If you can, start out with a slow jog to warm up the body.

<u>Heel raises</u> - stand facing a wall or fence. Place both hands on wall/fence for support and simply lift your heels so that you are standing on the balls of your feet. Lift and lower 10 times fairly quickly.

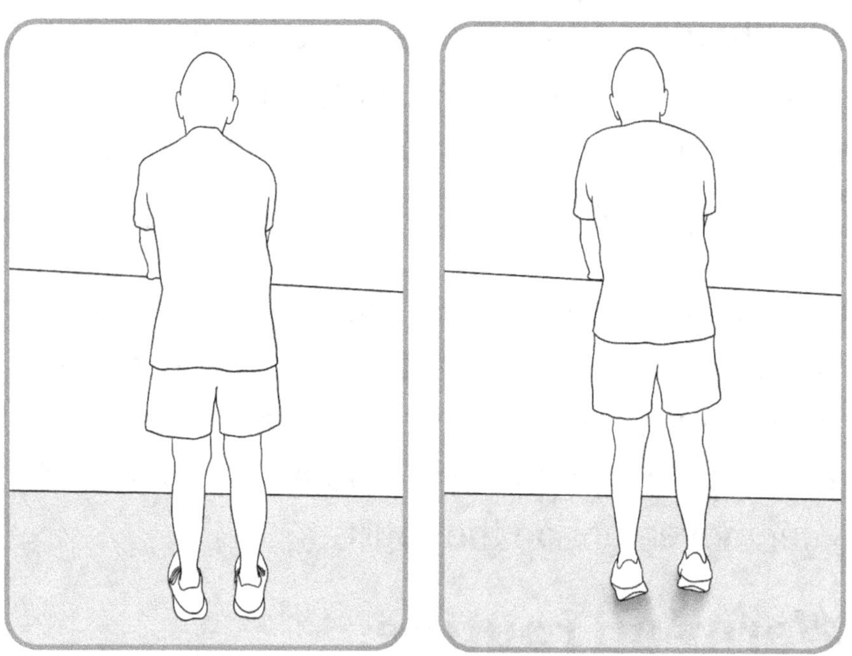

<u>Butt kicks</u> – stand parallel to a wall or fence. Place your hand closest to the wall/fence on the wall/fence for support. Standing with feet approximately shoulder width apart, keep your thigh and upper body vertical and bend your knee, lifting your heel up towards your butt, then lower your foot to the floor and repeat with the opposite leg. Do this 10 times, alternating sides.

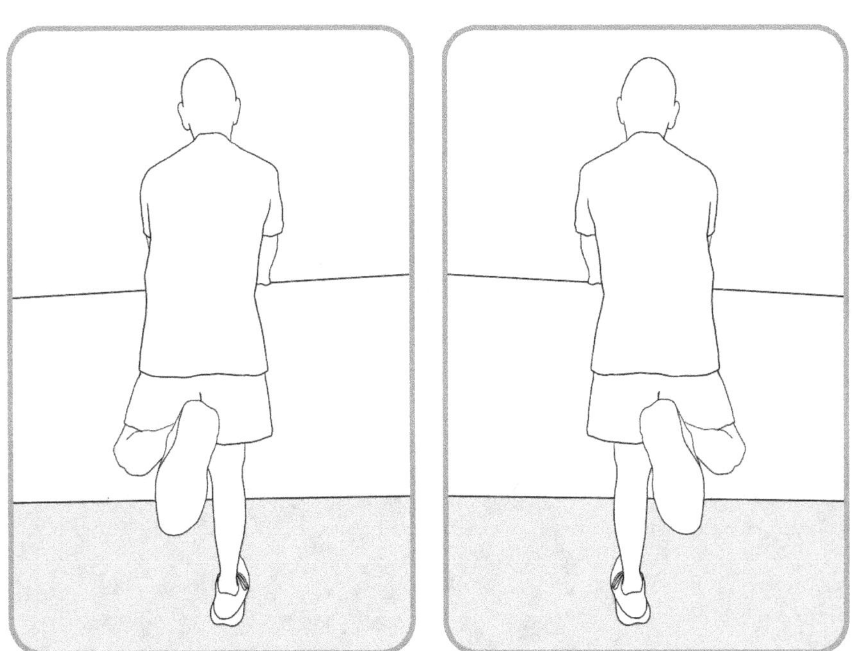

<u>Leg swings forward and back</u> - stand parallel to a wall or fence. Place your hand closest to the wall or fence on the wall/fence for support. Swing the opposite leg forward and back 10 times. Turn 180-degrees and repeat on the other leg.

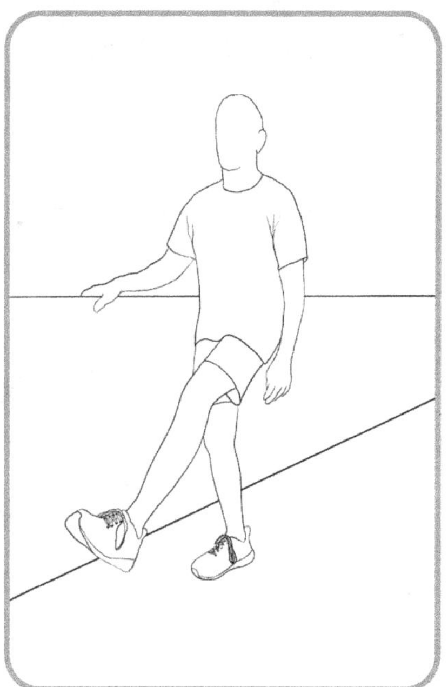
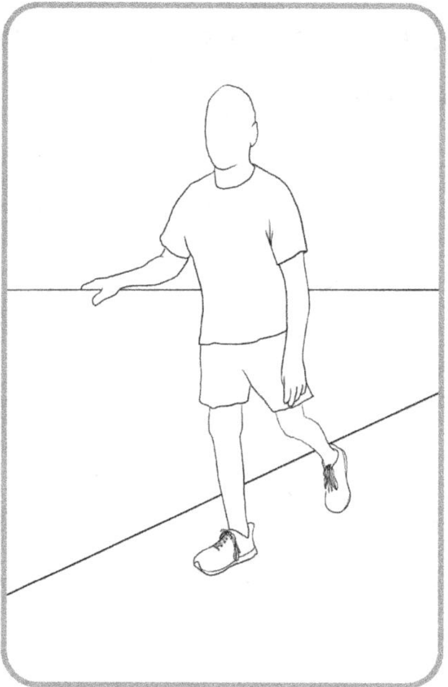

<u>Leg swings side to side</u> - stand facing the wall/ fence and place your hands on the wall/fence for balance. Swing your right leg across the front of your body, towards your left side, then swing it out to the right. Do this 10 times, then repeat with your left leg.

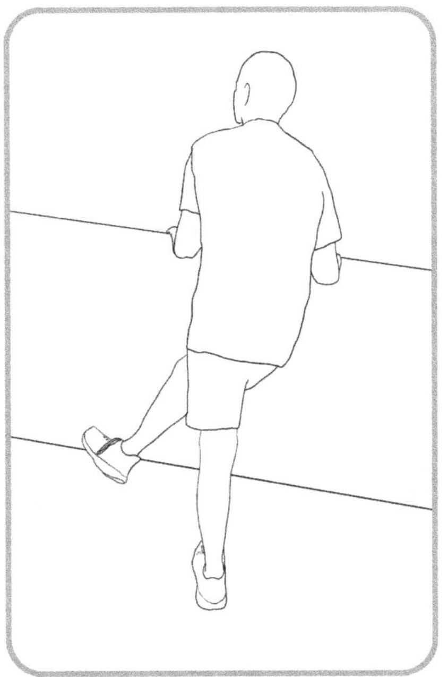
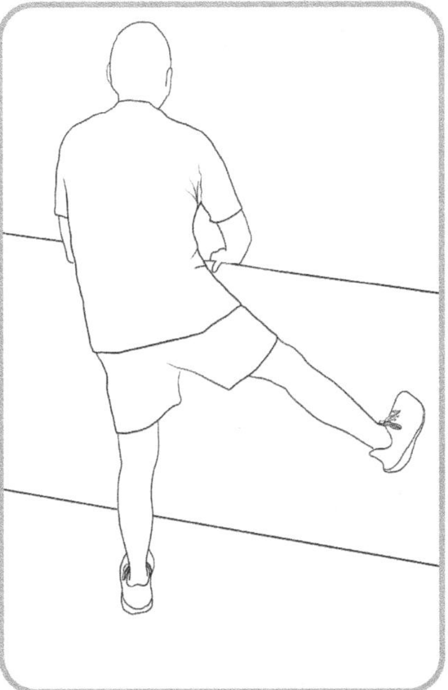

<u>**Hip circles**</u> - you've probably done arm swings to loosen up your arms and shoulders, well this is similar, only using your legs. Stand facing the wall/fence and place your hands on the wall/fence for balance. Starting with your right leg, rotate your leg/hip forward and make 10 circles forward, then reverse and make 10 circles backward. Repeat with your left leg.

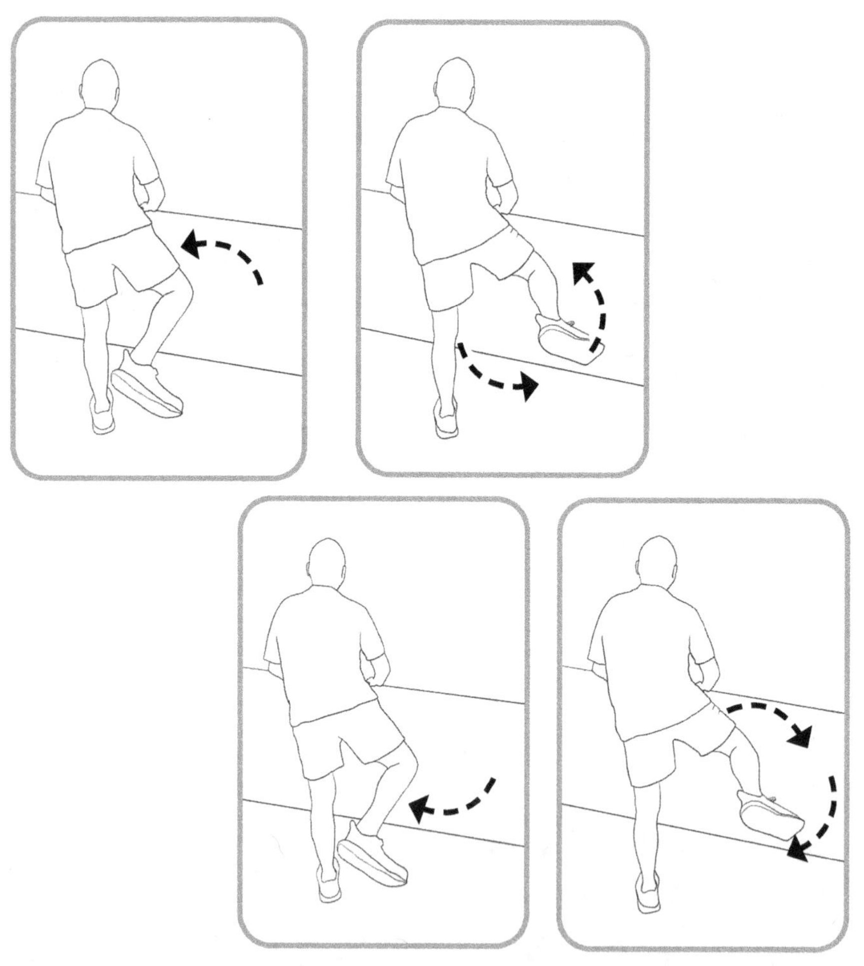

<u>March in Place</u> – Stand parallel to a wall or fence and place your hand closest to the wall/fence on the wall/fence for support. Lift knees alternately, 10 times with each leg.

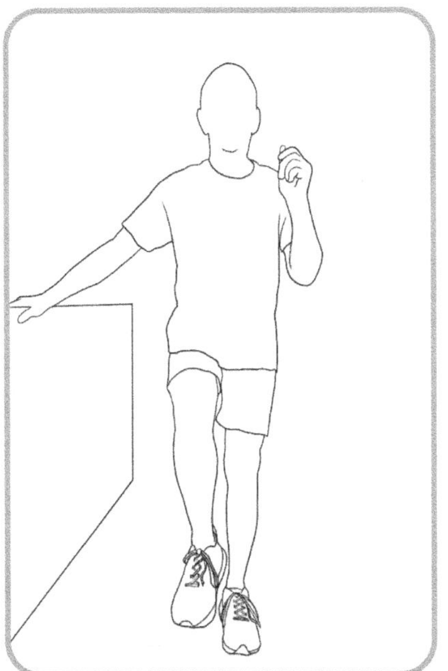 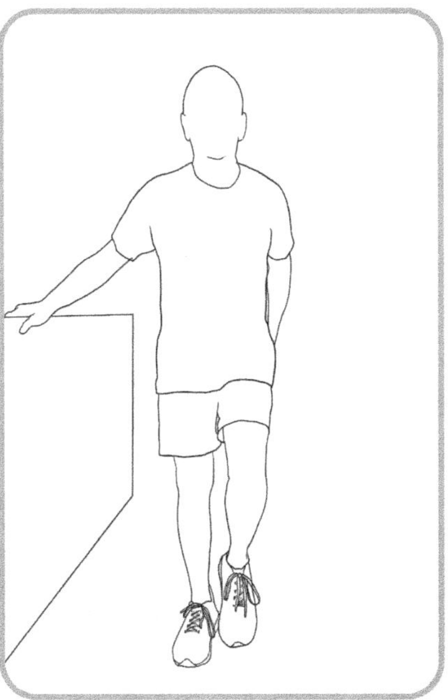

COOL DOWN

Okay, this is where those slow stretches come into play. An easy cool down stretch is to sit on a bench and twist your body to the right, bringing the outside of your right knee onto the bench, with your left foot on the ground, toes down and on the ball of your foot. Then place your elbows on the bench and hold the stretch for 30-60 seconds. Repeat on the other side.

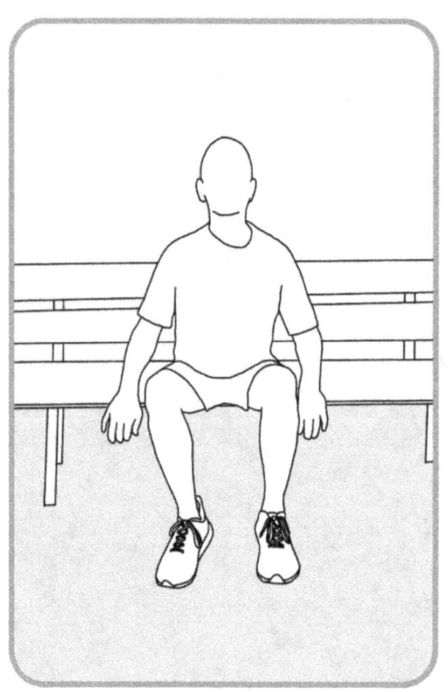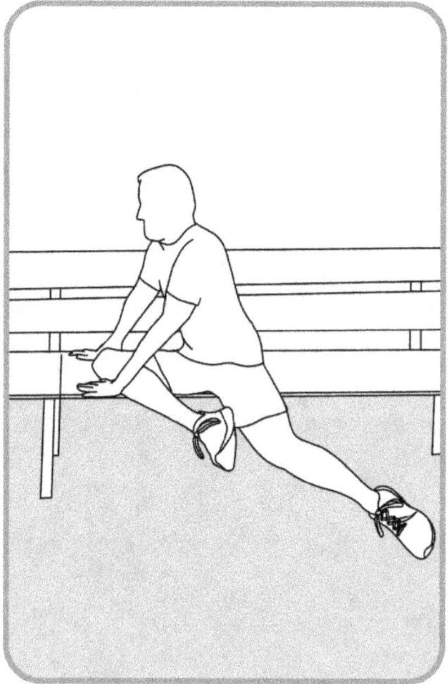

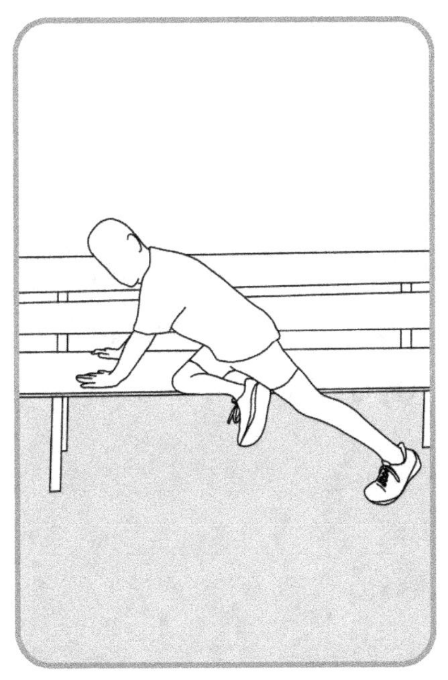 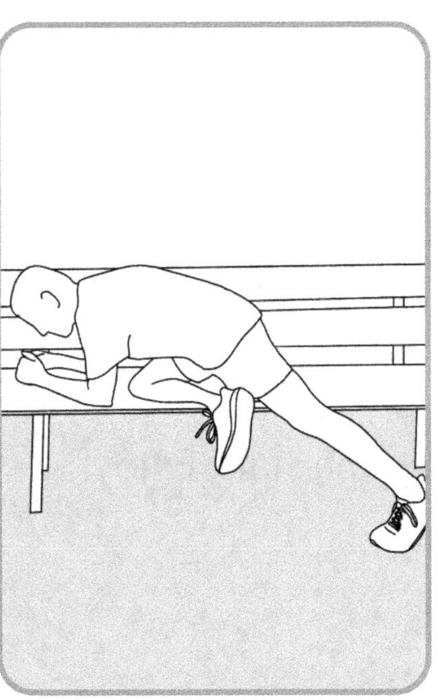

Now our hope is that you get out there and have some fun. Play the game, just be sure to listen to your doctor and therapist's advice and listen to your body. Do what you can to prepare it for the sport you are playing and listen when it let's you know it needs some attention. Remember, Our bodies have amazing abilities to overcome many physical, visual and emotional setbacks allowing us to enjoy returning to play a variety of sports and engaging in activities that restore our joy and sense of well-being.

David & Deborah Jeffrey

P.S. We've included a Pickleball journal on the following pages, so that you can log your game preparation, play, your body's response, and game stats. Enjoy!

Pickleball Journal

The purpose of this journal is to help you keep a dated record of the times you play pickleball and your positive recollections of your match.

- Did you show improvement in your serve placement and speed?

- After each serve did you quickly return to a ready stance, with knees slightly bent, slightly bent at the waist, body weight balanced on both feet, with knees slightly bent and feet apart to maximize balance?

- What aspects of your play need improvement?

- What were your physical abilities during the match?

- Did you feel off balance?

- Were you short of breath?

- Did your heart rate feel significantly increased?

All this information will help you create a plan on how to safely improve your pickleball play.

Remember to always play within your present physical fitness ability. If you feel excessively fatigued, let your opponents know that you need a break, and they can find a substitute to take your place. This will allow you to rest, enabling your body to recover and protecting you from over exertion and possible injury.

Our goal is to gradually improve our endurance, balance, understanding of the game, and most importantly enjoy the company of like-minded people embracing fun activity, while improving our fitness, health, and sense of well-being.

Date: _______________________________

	☺	😐	☹	
Today's Goals:				
PRE-GAME	☺	😐	☹	**Comments**
Mood				
Hydration				
Warm-up				
POST-GAME	☺	😐	☹	**Comments**
Serve placement				
Serve speed				
Ready stance				
Cool down				
PHYSICAL	☺	😐	☹	**Comments**
Balance				
Breathing				
Heart rate				
Endurance				
Other				

Things I did well:	Things to work on:

GAME STATS			
Where played			
Partner			
Games Won		Games Lost	

Date: _______________________

	🙂	😐	☹️	
Today's Goals:				
PRE-GAME	🙂	😐	☹️	**Comments**
Mood				
Hydration				
Warm-up				
POST-GAME	🙂	😐	☹️	**Comments**
Serve placement				
Serve speed				
Ready stance				
Cool down				
PHYSICAL	🙂	😐	☹️	**Comments**
Balance				
Breathing				
Heart rate				
Endurance				
Other				

Things I did well:	Things to work on:

GAME STATS			
Where played			
Partner			
Games Won		Games Lost	

Date: _______________________________

	🙂	😐	🙁	
Today's Goals:				
PRE-GAME	🙂	😐	🙁	**Comments**
Mood				
Hydration				
Warm-up				
POST-GAME	🙂	😐	🙁	**Comments**
Serve placement				
Serve speed				
Ready stance				
Cool down				
PHYSICAL	🙂	😐	🙁	**Comments**
Balance				
Breathing				
Heart rate				
Endurance				
Other				

Things I did well:	Things to work on:

GAME STATS	
Where played	
Partner	
Games Won	Games Lost

Date: _______________________________________

	🙂	😐	☹️	
Today's Goals:				
PRE-GAME	🙂	😐	☹️	**Comments**
Mood				
Hydration				
Warm-up				
POST-GAME	🙂	😐	☹️	**Comments**
Serve placement				
Serve speed				
Ready stance				
Cool down				
PHYSICAL	🙂	😐	☹️	**Comments**
Balance				
Breathing				
Heart rate				
Endurance				
Other				

Things I did well:	Things to work on:

GAME STATS			
Where played			
Partner			
Games Won		Games Lost	

Date: ______________________________

	😊	😐	☹️	
Today's Goals:				
PRE-GAME	😊	😐	☹️	**Comments**
Mood				
Hydration				
Warm-up				
POST-GAME	😊	😐	☹️	**Comments**
Serve placement				
Serve speed				
Ready stance				
Cool down				
PHYSICAL	😊	😐	☹️	**Comments**
Balance				
Breathing				
Heart rate				
Endurance				
Other				

Things I did well:	Things to work on:

GAME STATS			
Where played			
Partner			
Games Won		Games Lost	

Date: _______________________________

	🙂	😐	☹️	
Today's Goals:				

PRE-GAME	🙂	😐	☹️	Comments
Mood				
Hydration				
Warm-up				

POST-GAME	🙂	😐	☹️	Comments
Serve placement				
Serve speed				
Ready stance				
Cool down				

PHYSICAL	🙂	😐	☹️	Comments
Balance				
Breathing				
Heart rate				
Endurance				
Other				

Things I did well:	Things to work on:

GAME STATS	
Where played	
Partner	
Games Won	Games Lost

Date: _______________________________

	🙂	😐	🙁	Comments
Today's Goals:				
PRE-GAME	🙂	😐	🙁	**Comments**
Mood				
Hydration				
Warm-up				
POST-GAME	🙂	😐	🙁	**Comments**
Serve placement				
Serve speed				
Ready stance				
Cool down				
PHYSICAL	🙂	😐	🙁	**Comments**
Balance				
Breathing				
Heart rate				
Endurance				
Other				

Things I did well:	Things to work on:

GAME STATS		
Where played		
Partner		
Games Won		Games Lost

Date: ___________________________________

	🙂	😐	☹️	
Today's Goals:				
PRE-GAME	🙂	😐	☹️	**Comments**
Mood				
Hydration				
Warm-up				
POST-GAME	🙂	😐	☹️	**Comments**
Serve placement				
Serve speed				
Ready stance				
Cool down				
PHYSICAL	🙂	😐	☹️	**Comments**
Balance				
Breathing				
Heart rate				
Endurance				
Other				

Things I did well:	Things to work on:

GAME STATS			
Where played			
Partner			
Games Won		Games Lost	

Date: _______________________________

Today's Goals:				
PRE-GAME	☺	😐	☹	**Comments**
Mood				
Hydration				
Warm-up				
POST-GAME	☺	😐	☹	**Comments**
Serve placement				
Serve speed				
Ready stance				
Cool down				
PHYSICAL	☺	😐	☹	**Comments**
Balance				
Breathing				
Heart rate				
Endurance				
Other				

Things I did well:	Things to work on:

GAME STATS			
Where played			
Partner			
Games Won		Games Lost	

Date: _______________________________

Today's Goals:				
PRE-GAME	☺	😐	☹	**Comments**
Mood				
Hydration				
Warm-up				
POST-GAME	☺	😐	☹	**Comments**
Serve placement				
Serve speed				
Ready stance				
Cool down				
PHYSICAL	☺	😐	☹	**Comments**
Balance				
Breathing				
Heart rate				
Endurance				
Other				

Things I did well:	Things to work on:

GAME STATS			
Where played			
Partner			
Games Won		Games Lost	

Date: _______________________________

Today's Goals:				
PRE-GAME	🙂	😐	🙁	**Comments**
Mood				
Hydration				
Warm-up				
POST-GAME	🙂	😐	🙁	**Comments**
Serve placement				
Serve speed				
Ready stance				
Cool down				
PHYSICAL	🙂	😐	🙁	**Comments**
Balance				
Breathing				
Heart rate				
Endurance				
Other				

Things I did well:	Things to work on:

GAME STATS			
Where played			
Partner			
Games Won		Games Lost	

Date: _______________________________

Today's Goals:				
PRE-GAME	☺	😐	☹	**Comments**
Mood				
Hydration				
Warm-up				
POST-GAME	☺	😐	☹	**Comments**
Serve placement				
Serve speed				
Ready stance				
Cool down				
PHYSICAL	☺	😐	☹	**Comments**
Balance				
Breathing				
Heart rate				
Endurance				
Other				

Things I did well:	Things to work on:

GAME STATS			
Where played			
Partner			
Games Won		Games Lost	

Date: ___________________________________

	🙂	😐	☹️	
Today's Goals:				
PRE-GAME	🙂	😐	☹️	**Comments**
Mood				
Hydration				
Warm-up				
POST-GAME	🙂	😐	☹️	**Comments**
Serve placement				
Serve speed				
Ready stance				
Cool down				
PHYSICAL	🙂	😐	☹️	**Comments**
Balance				
Breathing				
Heart rate				
Endurance				
Other				

Things I did well:	Things to work on:

GAME STATS		
Where played		
Partner		
Games Won		Games Lost

Date: _______________________

	☺	😐	☹	Comments
Today's Goals:				
PRE-GAME	☺	😐	☹	**Comments**
Mood				
Hydration				
Warm-up				
POST-GAME	☺	😐	☹	**Comments**
Serve placement				
Serve speed				
Ready stance				
Cool down				
PHYSICAL	☺	😐	☹	**Comments**
Balance				
Breathing				
Heart rate				
Endurance				
Other				

Things I did well:	Things to work on:

GAME STATS	
Where played	
Partner	
Games Won	Games Lost

Date: _______________________________

Today's Goals:				

PRE-GAME	🙂	😐	🙁	**Comments**
Mood				
Hydration				
Warm-up				

POST-GAME	🙂	😐	🙁	**Comments**
Serve placement				
Serve speed				
Ready stance				
Cool down				

PHYSICAL	🙂	😐	🙁	**Comments**
Balance				
Breathing				
Heart rate				
Endurance				
Other				

Things I did well:	Things to work on:

GAME STATS	
Where played	
Partner	
Games Won	Games Lost

Date: _______________________________

	😀	😐	🙁	
Today's Goals:				
PRE-GAME	😀	😐	🙁	**Comments**
Mood				
Hydration				
Warm-up				
POST-GAME	😀	😐	🙁	**Comments**
Serve placement				
Serve speed				
Ready stance				
Cool down				
PHYSICAL	😀	😐	🙁	**Comments**
Balance				
Breathing				
Heart rate				
Endurance				
Other				

Things I did well:	Things to work on:

GAME STATS	
Where played	
Partner	
Games Won	Games Lost

Date: _______________________________

	☺	😐	☹	Comments
Today's Goals:				
PRE-GAME	☺	😐	☹	**Comments**
Mood				
Hydration				
Warm-up				
POST-GAME	☺	😐	☹	**Comments**
Serve placement				
Serve speed				
Ready stance				
Cool down				
PHYSICAL	☺	😐	☹	**Comments**
Balance				
Breathing				
Heart rate				
Endurance				
Other				

Things I did well:	Things to work on:

GAME STATS			
Where played			
Partner			
Games Won		Games Lost	

Date: ______________________________

	😊	😐	😞	
Today's Goals:				
PRE-GAME	😊	😐	😞	**Comments**
Mood				
Hydration				
Warm-up				
POST-GAME	😊	😐	😞	**Comments**
Serve placement				
Serve speed				
Ready stance				
Cool down				
PHYSICAL	😊	😐	😞	**Comments**
Balance				
Breathing				
Heart rate				
Endurance				
Other				

Things I did well:	Things to work on:

GAME STATS			
Where played			
Partner			
Games Won		Games Lost	

Date: _______________________

	🙂	😐	🙁	Comments
Today's Goals:				
PRE-GAME	🙂	😐	🙁	**Comments**
Mood				
Hydration				
Warm-up				
POST-GAME	🙂	😐	🙁	**Comments**
Serve placement				
Serve speed				
Ready stance				
Cool down				
PHYSICAL	🙂	😐	🙁	**Comments**
Balance				
Breathing				
Heart rate				
Endurance				
Other				

Things I did well:	Things to work on:

GAME STATS			
Where played			
Partner			
Games Won		Games Lost	

Date: ___________________________________

Today's Goals:	

PRE-GAME	🙂	😐	☹️	**Comments**
Mood				
Hydration				
Warm-up				

POST-GAME	🙂	😐	☹️	**Comments**
Serve placement				
Serve speed				
Ready stance				
Cool down				

PHYSICAL	🙂	😐	☹️	**Comments**
Balance				
Breathing				
Heart rate				
Endurance				
Other				

Things I did well:	Things to work on:

GAME STATS	
Where played	
Partner	
Games Won		Games Lost	

Date: _______________________________

	😊	😐	☹️	
Today's Goals:				
PRE-GAME	😊	😐	☹️	**Comments**
Mood				
Hydration				
Warm-up				
POST-GAME	😊	😐	☹️	**Comments**
Serve placement				
Serve speed				
Ready stance				
Cool down				
PHYSICAL	😊	😐	☹️	**Comments**
Balance				
Breathing				
Heart rate				
Endurance				
Other				

Things I did well:	Things to work on:

GAME STATS			
Where played			
Partner			
Games Won		Games Lost	

Date: _______________________________

	😊	😐	😞	
Today's Goals:				
PRE-GAME	😊	😐	😞	**Comments**
Mood				
Hydration				
Warm-up				
POST-GAME	😊	😐	😞	**Comments**
Serve placement				
Serve speed				
Ready stance				
Cool down				
PHYSICAL	😊	😐	😞	**Comments**
Balance				
Breathing				
Heart rate				
Endurance				
Other				

Things I did well:	Things to work on:

GAME STATS	
Where played	
Partner	
Games Won		Games Lost	

Date: _______________________

	🙂	😐	🙁	
Today's Goals:				
PRE-GAME	🙂	😐	🙁	**Comments**
Mood				
Hydration				
Warm-up				
POST-GAME	🙂	😐	🙁	**Comments**
Serve placement				
Serve speed				
Ready stance				
Cool down				
PHYSICAL	🙂	😐	🙁	**Comments**
Balance				
Breathing				
Heart rate				
Endurance				
Other				

Things I did well:	Things to work on:

GAME STATS			
Where played			
Partner			
Games Won		Games Lost	

Date: _______________________________

Today's Goals:				
PRE-GAME	🙂	😐	🙁	**Comments**
Mood				
Hydration				
Warm-up				
POST-GAME	🙂	😐	🙁	**Comments**
Serve placement				
Serve speed				
Ready stance				
Cool down				
PHYSICAL	🙂	😐	🙁	**Comments**
Balance				
Breathing				
Heart rate				
Endurance				
Other				

Things I did well:	Things to work on:

GAME STATS			
Where played			
Partner			
Games Won		Games Lost	

Date: ______________________________

Today's Goals:				
PRE-GAME	🙂	😐	☹️	**Comments**
Mood				
Hydration				
Warm-up				
POST-GAME	🙂	😐	☹️	**Comments**
Serve placement				
Serve speed				
Ready stance				
Cool down				
PHYSICAL	🙂	😐	☹️	**Comments**
Balance				
Breathing				
Heart rate				
Endurance				
Other				

Things I did well:	Things to work on:

GAME STATS			
Where played			
Partner			
Games Won		Games Lost	

Date: _______________________________________

	🙂	😐	☹️	
Today's Goals:				
PRE-GAME	🙂	😐	☹️	**Comments**
Mood				
Hydration				
Warm-up				
POST-GAME	🙂	😐	☹️	**Comments**
Serve placement				
Serve speed				
Ready stance				
Cool down				
PHYSICAL	🙂	😐	☹️	**Comments**
Balance				
Breathing				
Heart rate				
Endurance				
Other				

Things I did well:	Things to work on:

GAME STATS			
Where played			
Partner			
Games Won		Games Lost	

Date: _______________________

	☺	😐	☹	Comments
Today's Goals:				
PRE-GAME	☺	😐	☹	**Comments**
Mood				
Hydration				
Warm-up				
POST-GAME	☺	😐	☹	**Comments**
Serve placement				
Serve speed				
Ready stance				
Cool down				
PHYSICAL	☺	😐	☹	**Comments**
Balance				
Breathing				
Heart rate				
Endurance				
Other				

Things I did well:	Things to work on:

GAME STATS	
Where played	
Partner	
Games Won	Games Lost

Date: ______________________________

	😊	😐	☹️	
Today's Goals:				
PRE-GAME	😊	😐	☹️	**Comments**
Mood				
Hydration				
Warm-up				
POST-GAME	😊	😐	☹️	**Comments**
Serve placement				
Serve speed				
Ready stance				
Cool down				
PHYSICAL	😊	😐	☹️	**Comments**
Balance				
Breathing				
Heart rate				
Endurance				
Other				

Things I did well:	Things to work on:

GAME STATS	
Where played	
Partner	
Games Won	Games Lost

Date: _______________________________

	🙂	😐	🙁	
Today's Goals:				
PRE-GAME	🙂	😐	🙁	**Comments**
Mood				
Hydration				
Warm-up				
POST-GAME	🙂	😐	🙁	**Comments**
Serve placement				
Serve speed				
Ready stance				
Cool down				
PHYSICAL	🙂	😐	🙁	**Comments**
Balance				
Breathing				
Heart rate				
Endurance				
Other				

Things I did well:	Things to work on:

GAME STATS	
Where played	
Partner	
Games Won	Games Lost

Date: ___________________________

Today's Goals:	

PRE-GAME	🙂	😐	🙁	Comments
Mood				
Hydration				
Warm-up				

POST-GAME	🙂	😐	🙁	Comments
Serve placement				
Serve speed				
Ready stance				
Cool down				

PHYSICAL	🙂	😐	🙁	Comments
Balance				
Breathing				
Heart rate				
Endurance				
Other				

Things I did well:	Things to work on:

GAME STATS

Where played	
Partner	

Games Won		Games Lost	

Date: _______________________________

	☺	😐	☹	
Today's Goals:				
PRE-GAME	☺	😐	☹	**Comments**
Mood				
Hydration				
Warm-up				
POST-GAME	☺	😐	☹	**Comments**
Serve placement				
Serve speed				
Ready stance				
Cool down				
PHYSICAL	☺	😐	☹	**Comments**
Balance				
Breathing				
Heart rate				
Endurance				
Other				

Things I did well:	Things to work on:

GAME STATS			
Where played			
Partner			
Games Won		Games Lost	

Date: ____

Today's Goals:				
PRE-GAME	🙂	😐	🙁	**Comments**
Mood				
Hydration				
Warm-up				
POST-GAME	🙂	😐	🙁	**Comments**
Serve placement				
Serve speed				
Ready stance				
Cool down				
PHYSICAL	🙂	😐	🙁	**Comments**
Balance				
Breathing				
Heart rate				
Endurance				
Other				

Things I did well:	Things to work on:

GAME STATS			
Where played			
Partner			
Games Won		Games Lost	

If you enjoyed this book, we would appreciate it greatly if you left a positive review on Amazon.com.

For other Pickleball themed publications and products, please scan the following QR code, or visit www.debjeffrey.com/pickleball